R. J. HENNESSY

Surviving Motherhood

The Early Years of Parenthood: How to Stay Sane and Not Lose Your Shit

To my children...
Love, Mum xxx

Contents

1

Introduction: A bit about my journey into motherhood

You've probably picked up this book because you're a new mum or dad, maybe it was given to you as a gift or maybe you're one of my (mum) friends and had no choice but to read it… Just kidding… Anyways, I hope this book gives you some insight into my journey of motherhood and a reality of what some mothers will experience. I'm no perfect mother and there are days when I wish I was better (mum guilt is real…). I have no degree in child psychology or a job in childcare, just a book writing from experience which I hope you'll enjoy reading and maybe feel enlightened after.

A bit about me, I'm a mum of two which at the time of writing this they are 2 years old and a baby of 8 months. We also have a 4-year-old dog who has the best life in the house and doesn't know it. I was pregnant with my eldest during lock down. Back then I was grateful to be at home and no longer needing to travel. It gave me the time to rest and just enjoy the pregnancy. Everyone has a different story about their pregnancy, but I

1

loved it. I ate so much. I remember having two lunches one day just because at the time I was like, I'm eating for two! Looking back at it, I probably didn't need to eat that much and ended up working harder to lose the weight. There's so much pressure to look good and most of the new mums you see online or on TV look amazing. I always wondered how to these mums bounce back so quickly?! That was my first opinion of new mums, just bounce back and your back to your old self again…. Was a wrong, a bit about this later.

I wanted a home birth, not because of COVID and lock down but because of the fact you can only go into the labor ward once you were further along your labor. I wanted to be in the comforts of my own home, to feel relaxed. These were the things that would help me have an easy and smooth labor. The dog and the husband were great with providing oxytocin, the love hormone that you need when giving birth. Fortunately, I got all of that. I had the perfect home birth in a pool inside my baby's bedroom. It was around sunset and there was soft lighting. Yes, it truly was just magical. You don't get to hear many of these types of births as a lot of the time the media portrays such horrific births. There are indeed terrifying stories. So yes, very grateful. What did I do differently? I'm not sure, but I know reading a hypnobirthing book helped, taking a couple's workshop for pregnancy preparation and pregnancy yoga helped tremendously. I also made sure not to let myself get stressed about certain things. Stress is always there in our lives and it's just about managing that stress. Also, knowing I had lost my first pregnancy with a miscarriage, I made sure to take care of myself and took plenty of naps when I could.

So, for me, pregnancy and giving birth was the easiest. What came next was a complete shock to the system. If I could describe how my body felt soon after giving birth, it felt like I had been run over by a bus and that it decided to reverse and run back over me. The next few days and weeks were a whirlwind. I had this beautiful baby girl in my hands that filled our hearts with so much love, love I didn't think I even knew existed. At the same time, I was like, what the hell?! I'm shattered! You lose all focus on yourself and prioritise this tiny little baby that doesn't know anything else but the love you have and just how to cry. Oh, the crying and the waking up for feeds. If I could only just have a shower and sleep at the same time, then I'd feel like myself again. Do we ever feel like ourselves again? When we give birth to our child, we also give birth to motherhood.

Second pregnancy, not so easy when you have a 1.5year old toddler to run around after. There's no more enjoying that evening after work to put your feet up. Scrap that, you have a workout and another role to play – mum. Who needs the gym when you have a toddler. I enjoy exercise and find it's my time to be me again. This is my peace and quiet. I made sure to do postnatal Pilates. I needed that core strength and general strength exercise to keep up with the toddler. It was also important to stay physically strong postpartum. Not only do you have a small baby to lift but also a toddler to keep up with! I had a lot of false positives with test results too which after scans, further blood tests and an amniocentesis all turned out negative. This all happened in the few weeks leading to moving out the house. Very stressful times but somehow still managed to keep my cool with the toddler and work. We didn't move into our new home till nearly two months of temporary accommodation, but I did have that home birth I wanted again.

Maternity the second time round was completely different. I guess, I learnt from the first to rest more and enjoy those first few weeks/months relaxing and recovering. It was OK to sit and feed the baby and watch TV. I also had a toddler which luckily was in nursery. The challenge was splitting my time with a baby and an energetic toddler whilst sleep deprived. I also felt stronger the 2nd time round. I remember with my first baby, feeling so weak. Boy, do they make car seats heavy! I wouldn't recommend to anyone to take them out the car with a baby in it! Either let that baby sleep in the car and you have some time yourself or take the baby out into a carrier/ sling and go about your day. Oh, and prams! At the time of purchasing ours we had no idea what type we needed. If I was to go back and pick another it would be a very light one and not one that feels like a bus. When I have both children in it, its heavy!

A not so brief intro about me but hopefully this book will give you some insight into my experience of motherhood and maybe some things you can take away to help you find your calm in the chaos of it all. You should be able to read this book in under 2hrs, maybe less. Feel free to read from start to finish, otherwise find a topic you're interested in and go from there. Happy reading!

2

Reality of Motherhood: Expectations vs Reality

There is so much expected of mothers. What should be and shouldn't. Maybe you're a bit like me who is a perfectionist and wants the best. I've learnt over time to let go. To just surrender to certain things and to fight certain battles. I guess I've gotten older and wiser. Either way, it helped manage my own expectations. By doing so, come out less stressed from it all.

So here is a list of some parenting myths and my thoughts on them:

1. **You'll spoil the baby holding them too much:** Really?!? How can you spoil a baby when all they need is just endless love, cuddles, affection and doesn't know how to communicate other than crying. These small bundles of joy have been living inside you for nine months. Hold them close because one day they may not want you to hug

them. My toddler already doesn't want hugs from me, so enjoy that baby phase. Enjoy sitting on the sofa feeding them because once they start walking and talking, you'll look back and be missing those days. Your baby has had a very cosy cocoon growing inside you for the last nine months and now must live in this big world. They long for that closeness and warmth. Your smells, your voice, all soothing to a baby. Embrace them, they know nothing but instant love for you.

2. **Parenting comes naturally:** The number of times I have looked online to figure out why is my baby crying?! It could be anything - hunger, tiredness, teething or just wants to cry. Maybe it's a loud noise, maybe they are too cold/ hot. Parenting is hard. Both my parents weren't around for both my babies. Therefore, I have had to look elsewhere for some guidance. I guess using my own intuition a lot of the time and learning from how I was raised. The likes and dislikes have helped shape me become the parent I am today. With the second, I feel I've eased into parenthood and a lot more relaxed. They can cry a little bit longer so I can finish my cup of tea or go to the toilet. I've got the baby monitor on right now and can see the baby awake happily playing in his cot with his comforter. First time round, I would have rushed in as soon as I saw her wake and cry. Leaving them for a few mins is good for them.

3. **Your kids needs always come first:** It's a hard balance between time for yourself and your children. Especially in those early years. Naturally you will just focus on your baby and forget about yourself. I remember with my eldest, I would sign us up to loads of baby activities. This was to

just get out the house and in hope she would enjoy them. It turns out, if she saw I was enjoying them, then she would too. Swimming was our favorite and great for bonding. Second time round, I spent more time doing mother-baby fitness classes. It was great, as I really helped me get fit and make some new mum friends. Baby was also happy and content just watching me and other mums and babies. I feel it's good show your hobbies to your children like exercising. Happy mum, Happy baby.

4. **Going from none to one is harder than going from one to more:** As I mentioned before, parenting is hard (I'll mention this a lot in this book). It's probably the hardest thing I have done so far and I'm not one to shy away from a challenge. First time round, it's all new and a shock to the system. If you think you are a decisive person, (I like to think I am) you'll soon be questioning, is this right? Especially when there is a child screaming at you, you just can't think clearly. I remember the early months of my first born. Baby was fast asleep, maybe 4am and I had woken up with engorged breasts. My first thought was, do I wake the baby up and feed her? Do I let her sleep and pump? But then if I pump will I have enough milk in me for her if she wakes? Basically, you just lie there in bed wondering what to do. In the end, I just pumped one breast and as soon as I had finished, she woke and drank the other. When you have another child, you forget the shock of that newborn phase. No matter how close apart or far they are in age. You learn to be a new parent again, now a mum of 2 or etc.

5. **A good parent never shouts:** You will find some very stressful situations and will want to shout. You're releasing

your stress. Or maybe cry. I have cried plenty of times. The key thing is to talk through it after in a calm voice. Having children will test your relationship with your partner. No wonder so many relationships fail after having kids. You are no longer just the two of you. You no longer have that time for each other, you'll have to make up that time. There are times when I have been so exhausted from not having a moment to myself and then it takes one thing (it could be anything) and you just lose your shit. I have had to just walk away. When the husband wants to talk, I'm too tired to say anything. Or maybe too angry. So, I don't, as sometimes just keeping quiet is better than to say something unkind. Yes, it is OK to shout. Just step back, take a deep breath, maybe a few deep breaths and just start again fresh.

Those are my 5. I'm sure there are plenty. Maybe you have heard a few yourself? How do those make you feel. Remember they are just myths. You can interpretate them however you like, just don't lose your mind over them and if you do, just let it go. Focus on the things that are important to you.

3

In the beginning – Pregnancy

As mentioned previously, I planned for a homebirth and was able to have just that. If you are currently pregnant reading this book, then enjoy it. Both my pregnancies were different to each other. In my first, the first trimester I had awful skin. My eczema just went crazy, and I'd react to everything. I kept thinking, aren't you supposed to be glowing when you're pregnant? I wasn't, at least for those first two trimesters. The last trimester, my skin started to glow, but I had awful back pains. I could not sit on the sofa and had to sit on one of those pregnancy/Pilates ball every time. Oh, and sleep! How are you supposed to sleep with this massage bump growing. You're supposed to sleep on your left side which I found extremely difficult as I had pains on my left side and ended up just sleeping on my right. I know mums who are front sleepers. That must have taken some time to get used to. They say to get as much rest when you are pregnant, and you should because motherhood is very demanding. It's a marathon. I loved napping. The pregnancy takes a lot out of you. A baby is growing inside of you and taking all those good nutrients. It's going to wear you out. Napping during pregnancy felt easier. I remember just being able to lie down and close my eyes and I was gone instantly. Completely different now after baby arrives. There's that horrible feeling that as soon as you close your eyes and fall asleep, your baby will wake up. It's awful. No wonder why so many women suffer from insomnia.

Second pregnancy, I was more tired and a nauseous in the first trimester. I hear stories of plenty of mums being sick, some even having to take medication. It's awful, what we must go through to bring life into this world. Second time pregnancy, my back wasn't as weak. I was able to sit on the sofa this time. I didn't have as many cravings and wasn't stuffing my face as much. If you can guess, my first I had a girl and second a boy. They say that a baby girl takes away the mother's beauty. Well, I was glowing more the second time round!

Preparation for Labor

Throughout both pregnancies, I did pregnancy yoga classes and practiced hypnobirthing which prepared me for the birth of my babies. Here are some useful tips for getting ready for labor and birth:

1. Take childbirth classes – these can prepare you for what to expect during labor i.e. when you'll need to go into hospital or labor ward or call your midwife and the difference with Braxton hicks.
2. Birth Plan – share this with your partner and midwife. Lab our can be unpredictable, so it's always good to write

down your preferences. Especially as when it gets to the big day you may not want to talk to anyone. So, whether is dim lighting, soft playing music, no talking etc. Write it all down.

3. Get a good playlist. I found just having some good tunes to listen to throughout my pregnancy helped me to relax. Also nice to have these tunes playing whilst you are in labor. Once the baby arrives, you'll find these tunes help keep you and the baby calm during those stressful moments.

4. Practice relaxation techniques. I found listening to positive labor affirmations helped. You can find a few on Spotify or if you've been taken hypnobirthing classes, you may have some prerecording's from the instructor. I found pregnancy yoga very helpful.

5. Pack your hospital bag. Only 5% of babies arrive on their due date so be prepared for that day. For my first pregnancy I hadn't one packed as I was so confident that I would have the baby at home. Luckily, I didn't need one but the second time round I did have one pack. Here are some essential items to pack in your bag:

- Nightgown
- Heavy duty maternity pads – you will be bleeding a lot after birth.
- Underwear
- Bra's – nursing ones if you want to breastfeed.
- Toiletries
- Phone and charger.
- Clothes
- Snacks and drinks
- Entertainment – book, tablet, or personal music

Preparation for Baby

1. Get your baby essential list ready. Here's mine:
2. Newborn nappies and wet wipes
3. Bed side crib (you can get the nursery crib post baby if you want as they won't need to sleep in it till after 6 months)
4. Newborn instant formula – your milk will take a few days before your milk supply to come in as you'll initially have colostrum. So, it's always good to have this handy.
5. Newborn clothes and hat – I remember the first time I unfolded my baby's clothes and placed them on my belly thinking this baby is so tiny and getting so excited to meet them!
6. Car seat – these things are heavy beasts and feel even heavier after you've given birth. I suggest going to the shops to have a good luck before deciding on one that suits.
7. Pram – Find one that will suit your lifestyle.
8. Nursing pillow - I bought a pregnancy pillow which could also be used as a nursing one. Baby stuff takes up a lot of room. So, if you have limited space, then be smart about what you buy as your home will soon feel very small.
9. Muslin clothes – to wipe up any spills including vomit.
10. Blanket
11. Sling or Carrier – that newborn phase they just want to be held.
12. Breast Pump if you are feeding and want to express.
13. Bottles and Steriliser – you can buy bottles that sterilise in the microwave. So, save yourself some space and get those!
14. Newborn Bath insert/ Bath

There are more items that you can get but these are my main ones that will help you initially. You'll find that you end up buying so many things or if you are lucky enough get handed down items. Some of these you won't even need. I feel, if you get the basics, you'll find a way to get round.

1. Meal preparation – get those batch cooking recipes and start freezing them. You'll need those quick meals that you can just throw in the oven or microwave. If you don't enjoy cooking, then get those ready-made ones. You can find some healthy ones available and some companies even give you discounts for new parents.
2. Prepare siblings. I found reading books about being a big sister or there being a baby growing inside me helpful.

Fun Things to do before the baby arrives.

1. Go on a babymoon. Unfortunately, due to COVID we never went on one with the first pregnancy. We did with the second one but going on holiday heavily pregnant with a toddler isn't so much a holiday. So go before you get too uncomfortable!
2. Pamper yourself. I love a massage and you can find some good pregnancy massages. Get yourself a good facial and your nails done!
3. Find a parenting community. We signed up to NCT and so lucky with the mum and dads to be we met. Our babies were all born around the same age and these mums helped me get through motherhood. They say you need a village to raise a family. Find your village!

4. Have a date night. You don't know when you're going to get your next one!
5. Decorate the nursery together. This was fun!
6. Attend your baby shower. For both my pregnancies they were both surprises. Unfortunately for my second I was so ill that I didn't turn up to it!

4

The Birth

You have the right to choose how you want to give birth. The type of birth depends on your baby's health, your preferences and where. Your midwife will be the best person to speak to about the pros and cons of giving birth vaginally or c-section. If any complications arise you may be offered an induction or a C-section. The NHS offers an induction if you don't go into labor before 41 weeks as this reduces the risk of still birth and complications. A very useful tool to help decide regarding the birth of your baby is to use the B.R.A.I.N acronym.

B – Benefits
What are the benefits of having this procedure or intervention?

R – Risks
What are the risks to me and the baby and how will it affect my labor and birth?

A – Alternatives

Are there alternatives? Can a different procedure be done instead?

I – Instinct

What are your instincts telling you? What feels right for you?

N – Nothing

What happens if I do nothing?

I found this very useful when I was advised not to have a homebirth due to the small fibroid I had. I was told I was at risk of postpartum hemorrhaging. Obviously with my science brain on, I did some research and found that mine were small in comparison and lower risk. Also speaking with my midwife, she advised me that she'd labored many women with fibroids. That they also carried oxytocin with them if it did happen. I also knew that worst case, I was less than a 10min drive from the hospital. It's always good to talk about your options and think it through. Do what feels right for you and your baby. Don't ever do anything you feel uncomfortable doing. Keep yourself well informed and do your research.

I was four days overdue with my first and remember being offered an induction. I reminded myself that the baby will arrive when it's ready. On my due date I went for a very long walk. Now it was mid-June, so you can imagine hot it was. Particularly, that summer. Heat and pregnancy are not a good combination. Imagine wearing a hot water bottle. That's exactly it…. Uncomfortable. I had a few days of Braxton hicks' contractions and then finally on the day I gave birth, I felt them.

The baby did some strange movement and knew that day was going to be day. My labor was very first and for a first-time mum giving birth, it was very smooth. Maybe it's the yoga teacher in me. I am sure there are other positive stories out there. We just don't hear much about them. They do exist!

The one thing I do remember after giving birth is the contractions to push the placenta out! You're already shattered, and you still have to push?! Yes, but you can get drugs for this. I decided I want to be drug free, except gas an air. Although, the mid-wife arrived 30mins before I gave birth so only really had it for 10mins. I'm not even sure if it made a difference at that point!

5

After Birth

Your recovery period can vary depending on how you delivered i.e. if you had a cesarean or pushed only 20 mins or were in labor for over 40 hours. Here's a timeline of how you'll feel:

Week 1

- Vaginal birth – physical status – vaginal will hurt depending on how much your perineum tore (this is the skin between your vagina and anus). You will be bleeding; this is normal. You should be wearing maternity pads as normal pads won't do the trick. Your uterus will begin to contract back to its original size. Breastfeeding also aids this.
- C- Section – physical status - Movement will be very difficult. The incision can be painful. Movement is recommended to avoid any blood clots. If a bladder catheter is used, it will be removed.
- Mental Status – Exhaustion. As I said earlier, like a bus running over you and reversing back to do it again. You'll

feel overwhelmed. Your hormones will be all over the place. Expect to cry or feeling like crying. It's OK, in fact do it, you'll feel better for doing so. You'll feel a tremendous amount of love for your baby. Even if you don't feel it instantly, that's normal too. You've been through a lot and may have had a traumatic birth.

Now after having my second one, I'm always amazed by how much my heart has grown for the love. I didn't think it was possible. But it does, it just feels bigger. I was always worried about whether there would be enough space to love more. But it's not space, it just grows. Metaphorically obviously.

Week 6

- Vaginal birth – Physical status - Uterus will return to its pre-pregnancy size. The bleeding stops but can potentially return. Most people are cleared for sexual activity and exercise.
- C- Section – Physical status. Same as vaginal. Just take things slow. Clear to drive and lift something other than your baby. The scar my feel numb or itchy.
- Mental Status – feeling overwhelmed and exhausted is normal. If you do feel deeper feelings about depression or anxiety, then discuss this with your doctor.

6 months

- Vaginal Birth – Physical status – if your hair was falling out, it should stop now. If you had issues with bladder control, then this shouldn't be an issue by 6 months. Make sure to continue with your pelvic floor exercising. Your period should have returned if not a year.

- C- Section – physical status – like above.
- Mental status – You may start to feel more like yourself here if your baby is starting to sleep for longer. I didn't. My second was still waking up every 3hrs. He only turned the corner close to 7 months.

One year

- Vaginal birth – you may feel like your own self again, but your body may still feel different and have gained some extra weight. Don't worry this is normal. I'm still trying to accept this myself and find this bit the hardest. Love the body you have.
- C-section – Your scar may have faded but may still feel a bit numb.
- Mental health status – You're probably feeling a lot more confident as a mother and getting used to motherhood. I would nap when you still can

6

Feeding

Breastfeeding

This is when you feed your baby breastmilk. I remember the first time doing it and were my nipples sore! Like you had to go through labour and now this!? Both my babies had tongue ties too. A condition which makes it difficult for babies to latch on and suck. You can get nipple guards, but I decided to persist. Eventually they do start becoming like bullets and you get used to it. The soreness does eventually go. Plenty of nipple balm helps. I've also tried cabbage leaves. They contain a natural chemical which helps sooth your nipples.

It's recommended to breastfeed your baby up to 6months. How often you breastfeed your baby will depend on your baby. Whether they want shorter frequent feeds or longer ones. Both my babies were breastfed, and both have different patterns. It's true, no two babies are the same. How often to feed your baby will also change as time goes. Newborns will feed every 2-3 hours can go through cluster feeding. When this happens make sure you are sitting somewhere comfortably and have a good show to watch!

Formula feeding

This is where you introduce formula to your baby through a bottle. Baby milk formula has as the nutrients needed for a baby. It is manufactured milk made for babies. With this, there is prep work required to formula feed. You'll need to make sure that the bottles are properly sterilised.

Some mothers also choose to pump their milk and feed this through a bottle to their babies.

There are pros and cons of doing both. I suggest do the one that suits you and your baby.

For both my babies, I introduced the bottle and found this helpful to get the dad involved and give me a break when I needed it. Babies are demanding, so it's important you find some me time when you can. I did attempt pumping but found this extra work on top of everything else. Again, do what suits you.

7

Self-Care isn't Selfish

ike I mentioned, motherhood is hard. It's important to find some time to yourself. In those first few months just so I could get more than 2-3 hours of sleep, I'd let my husband feed the baby so that I could sleep and then I would do the night shift. It did mean I would get 3-4hrs but it's better than 2hrs. If you have family around, then don't feel afraid to ask for help or get help if you can afford it. Whether that's someone watching the baby for 30mins so you can have a shower. Having a shower is the one thing in my day that I make sure I have. It's the one thing that makes me feel a little bit normal. What's yours? If you can do that one thing in your day, then you're doing ok. If you can't then you still are doing OK. Take each day as it comes. You're hear reading this book, which means you managed to find a moment to yourself even if its reading up something on motherhood.

I find physical exercise as my go to for endorphins and just to generally feel like myself again. When you have the go ahead from your doctor to exercise and feel up for it, then I highly recommend it. There are now plenty of postnatal classes out there. Even if you're not a gym-goer, a walk with the baby in a pram or sling will still make you feel good. Maybe you've made some mum friends in your antenatal classes. Start organising activities with them. If you haven't start joining some baby classes. You'll be surprised how many other mums you'll easily be able to connect with and share your baby stories with. It's important to connect as it can feel really isolating at times.

Just some activities I would do to get me out the house and away from chores:

- Baby sensory classes
- Music classes
- Baby swimming
- Buggy fitness classes
- Organised pram walks
- Postnatal Pilates with baby
- Baby massage classes
- Baby and mum yoga classes
- Baby reading classes.
- Baby sign language

I've made some new mum friends even with my second child and find these are the people that keep me sane. These are my saviours especially on those days when you feel the worst. Just turn up to your baby class. Whether you are late, you'll feel better for it. I've turned up a whole later late once thinking it started at that hour!

One thing I remember in the beginning is finding the time

to feed myself or the energy to cook and eat. Those batch cooked meals make a huge difference. Especially if you've been breastfeeding, I found I was always hungry. I would have a snack drawer filled with all sorts of snacks – cashew nuts, raisins, chocolates, and biscuits. My husband would make me smoothies in the morning just to get something quick and nutritious into me in. If you have toddler, you'll also soon realise that you'll end up eating their leftovers. I'm basically a human dust bin. I should just throw the food away but I just can't help throwing food. No wonder we mama's find it hard to shake off that extra weight.

Another important note is keeping the flame alive in your relationship. Being a parent is hard and your kids will take up a lot of you and your partner's time. By the end of the day, you're both shattered and have no energy left for each other. Spending time with your partner doesn't have to be another thing to do on your to-do list, it can help strengthen your relationship.

Some simple steps to have a more loving relationship with children:

- Set some time aside to talk about your goals and dreams as a couple.
- Just remember, you're in this for the long haul.
- Always share your thoughts and feelings often
- Turn off the TV – just spend some time together.
- Find a hobby or interest you both share. If you already have one, then great!
- Try to reminisce about those feeling you had for your partner before you met them. Try doing this when you

are doing a house chore like the washing up.
- Learn to let go…
- Remember that no family is perfect.
- Find something special in the ordinary tasks you have.
- Remember to be kind to one another. Be nice and loving

$$8$$

Conclusion: Reflecting and Celebrating

arenthood is hard, I've said this many times. Sometimes I feel like life has been sucked out of me. Especially on days when I have had little sleep. Either way, I wouldn't change it for the world. I have grown as a person and grateful for the family I have. Motherhood isn't about perfection. It's a learning journey. A marathon. One that is filled with love. Remember to celebrate your successes. Acknowledge the hard work and victories. Embrace the future challenges with confidence. Stay grounded. Keep the lessons learned close to heart.

I hope you have enjoyed reading this book and found it insightful. I would really appreciate it if you could leave a complimentary review on Amazon!

9

Resources

Crow, S. (2019, July 10). 17 Parenting myths people have believed for decades. Best Life. https://bestlife online.com/parenting-myths/

What are some common parenting myths to avoid? (n.d.). ABC Quality. https://abcquality.org/blog/what-are-some-common -parenting-myths-to-avoid/

Pampers. (2024, March 17). Preparing for Baby: 21 things to do Before Giving Birth. Web-Pampers-US-EN. https://www.p ampers.com/en-us/pregnancy/preparing-for-your-new-baby/ article/how-to-prepare-for-a-baby

Website, N. (2023, May 17). Your body after the birth. nhs.uk. https://www.nhs.uk/pregnancy/labour-and-birth/after-the-b irth/your-body/

Rasminsky, A. (2018, July 31). Your guide to postpartum

recovery. Healthline. https://www.healthline.com/health/postpartum-recovery-timeline#one-year

10 tips for keeping your relationship strong while raising kids. (2020, November 13). Gundersen Health System. https://www.gundersenhealth.org/health-wellness/pregnancy-kids/10-tips-for-keeping-your-relationship-strong-while-raising-kids#:~:text=Be%20nice%20and%20loving%20to,how%20to%20truly%20thank%20them.